The Ultimate Lean & Green Breakfast And Salad Cookbook

Delicious Lean & Green Breakfast And Salad Recipes For Beginners

Jesse Cohen

1

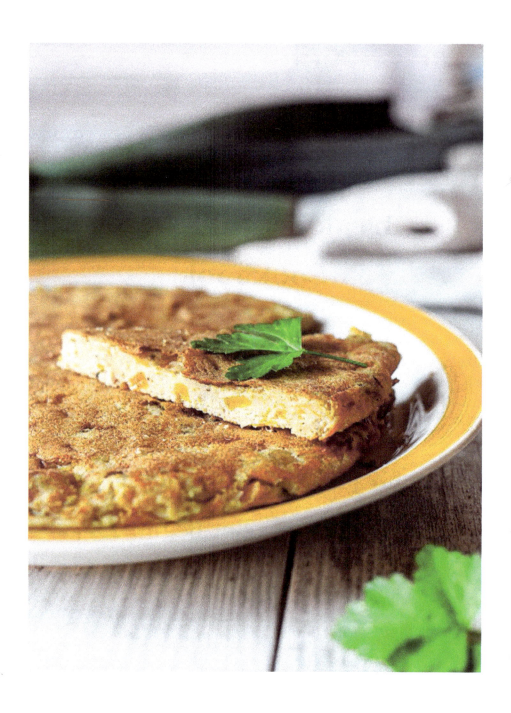

Table of contents

Avocado Toast

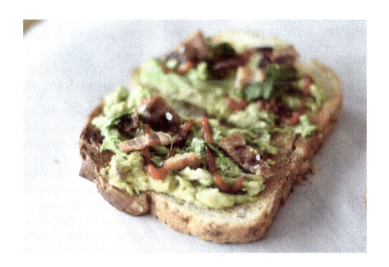

Servings: 4

Preparation Time: 15 minutes

Cooking Time: 4 minutes

Ingredients:

- 1 large avocado, peeled, pitted, and chopped roughly
- ¼ teaspoon of fresh lemon juice
- Salt and ground black pepper, as required
- 4 whole-wheat bread slices
- 4 hard-boiled eggs, peeled and sliced

Instructions:

1. In a bowl, add the avocado, and with a fork, mash roughly.

2. Add the lemon juice, salt, and black pepper and mix well and put aside.

3. Heat a non-stick frying pan on medium-high heat and toast the slice for about 2 minutes per side.

4. Repeat with the remaining slices.

5. Spread the avocado mixture over each slice evenly.

6. Top each with egg slices and serve immediately.

Baked Eggs

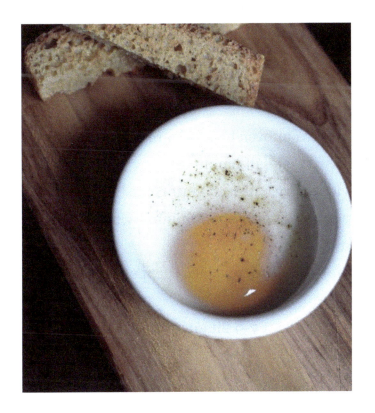

Servings: 6

Preparation Time: 10 minutes

Cooking Time: 9 minutes

Ingredients:

- 2 cups of fresh spinach, chopped finely
- 12 large eggs

- ½ cup of heavy cream
- ¾ cup of low-fat Parmesan cheese, shredded
- Salt and ground black pepper, as required

Instructions:

1. Preheat your oven to 425 degrees F.
2. Grease 12 cups of muffin tin.
3. Divide spinach in each muffin cup.
4. Crack an egg over spinach into each cup and drizzle with heavy cream.
5. Sprinkle with salt and black pepper, followed by Parmesan cheese.
6. Bake for about 7-9 minutes or until the desired doneness of eggs.
7. Serve immediately.

Eggs in Bell Pepper Rings

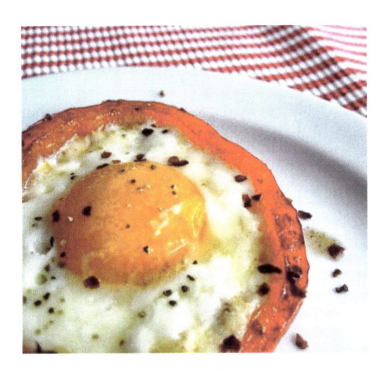

Servings: 2

Preparation Time: 10 minutes

Cooking Time: 6 minutes

Ingredients:

- 1 bell pepper, seeded and cut into 4 (¼-inch) rings
- 4 eggs
- Salt and ground black pepper, as required

- 1 tablespoon of fresh parsley, chopped
- 1 tablespoon of fresh chives, chopped

Instructions:

1. Heat a lightly greased non-stick skillet over medium heat.
2. Place 4 bell pepper rings in the skillet and cook for about 2 minutes.
3. Carefully flip the rings.
4. Crack an egg in the middle of every bell pepper ring and sprinkle with salt and black pepper.
5. Cook for about 2-4 minutes or until the desired doneness of eggs.
6. Carefully transfer the bell pepper rings to the serving plates and serve with parsley and chives' garnishing.

Eggs in Avocado Halves

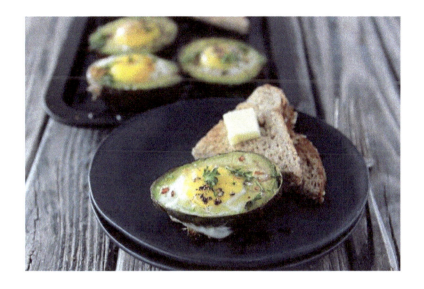

Servings: 2

Preparation Time: 10 minutes

Cooking Time: 15 minutes

Ingredients:

- 1 avocado, halved and pitted
- 2 eggs
- Salt and ground black pepper, as required
- ¼ cup of cherry tomatoes halved
- 2 cups of fresh baby spinach

Instructions:

1. Preheat your oven to 425 degrees F.
2. Carefully remove about 2 tablespoons of flesh from each avocado half.
3. Place avocado halves into a little baking dish.
4. Carefully crack an egg in each avocado half and sprinkle with salt and black pepper.
5. Bake for about 15 minutes or until the desired doneness of the eggs.
6. Arrange 1 avocado half onto each serving plate and serve alongside the cherry tomatoes and spinach.

Chicken & Zucchini Pancakes

Servings: 4

Preparation Time: 15 minutes

Cooking Time: 32 minutes

Ingredients:

- 4 cups of zucchinis, shredded
- Salt, as required
- ¼ cup of cooked chicken, shredded
- ¼ cup of scallion, chopped finely
- 1 egg, beaten
- ¼ cup of coconut flour
- Salt and ground black pepper, as required
- 1 tablespoon of extra-virgin olive oil

Instructions:

1. In a colander, place the zucchini and sprinkle with salt.
2. Put aside for about 8-10 minutes.
3. Squeeze the zucchinis well and transfer into a bowl.
4. In the bowl of zucchini, add the remaining ingredients and blend until well combined.
5. In a large non-stick skillet, heat the oil over medium heat.

6. Add ¼ cup of zucchini mixture into the preheated skillet and spread in a good layer.
7. Cook for about 3-4 minutes per side.
8. Repeat with the remaining mixture.
9. Serve warm.

Broccoli Waffles

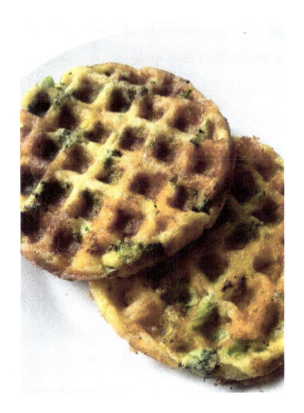

Servings: 2

Preparation Time: 10 minutes

Cooking Time: 8 minutes

Ingredients:

- 1/3 cup of broccoli, chopped finely
- ¼ cup of low-fat Cheddar cheese, shredded

- 1 egg
- ½ teaspoon of garlic powder
- ½ teaspoon of dried onion, minced
- Salt and ground black pepper, as required

Instructions:

1. Preheat a mini waffle iron, then grease it.
2. In a medium bowl, place all ingredients and blend until well combined.
3. Place ½ of the mixture into preheated waffle iron and cook for about 3-4 minutes or until golden brown.
4. Repeat with the remaining mixture.
5. Serve warm.

Cheesy Spinach Waffles

Servings: 4

Preparation Time: 10 minutes

Cooking Time: 20 minutes

Ingredients:

- 1 large egg, beaten
- 1 cup of ricotta cheese, crumbled
- ½ cup of part-skim mozzarella cheese, shredded
- ¼ cup of low-fat Parmesan cheese, grated
- 4 ounces of frozen spinach, thawed and squeezed dry
- 1 garlic clove, minced
- Salt and ground black pepper, as required

Instructions:

1. Preheat a mini waffle iron, then grease it.
2. In a bowl, add all the ingredients and beat until well combined.
3. Place ¼ of the mixture into preheated waffle iron and cook for about 4-5 minutes or until golden brown.
4. Repeat with the remaining mixture.
5. Serve warm.

Kale Scramble

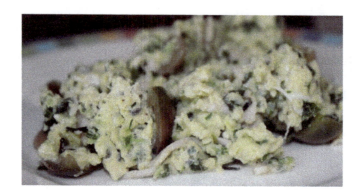

Servings: 2

Preparation Time: 10 minutes

Cooking Time: 6 minutes

Ingredients:

- 4 eggs
- 1/8 teaspoon of ground turmeric
- 1/8 teaspoon of red pepper flakes, crushed
- Salt and ground black pepper, as required
- 1 tablespoon of water
- 2 teaspoons of olive oil
- 1 cup of fresh kale, tough ribs removed, and chopped

Instructions:

1. In a bowl, add the eggs, turmeric, red pepper flakes, salt, black pepper, and water and with a whisk, beat until foamy.
2. In a skillet, heat the oil over medium heat
3. Add the egg mixture and stir to mix.
4. Immediately reduce the heat to medium-low and cook for about 1-2 minutes, stirring frequently.
5. Stir in the kale and cook for about 3-4 minutes, stirring frequently.
6. Remove from the heat and serve immediately.

Tomato & Egg Scramble

Servings: 2

Preparation Time: 10 minutes

Cooking Time: 5 minutes

Ingredients:

- 4 eggs
- ¼ teaspoon of red pepper flakes, crushed
- Salt and ground black pepper, as required
- ¼ cup of fresh basil, chopped
- ½ cup of tomatoes, chopped
- 1 tablespoon of olive oil

Instructions:

1. In a large bowl, add eggs, red pepper flakes, salt, and black pepper and beat well.
2. Add the basil and tomatoes and stir to mix.
3. In a large non-stick skillet, heat the oil over medium-high heat.
4. Add the egg mixture and cook for about 3-5 minutes, stirring continuously.
5. Serve immediately.

Tofu & Spinach Scramble

Servings: 2

Preparation Time: 10 minutes

Cooking Time: 8 minutes

Ingredients:

- 1 tablespoon of olive oil
- 1 garlic clove, minced
- ¼ pound medium-firm tofu, drained, pressed, and crumbled
- 1/3 cup of low-sodium vegetable broth
- 2¾ cups of fresh baby spinach
- 2 teaspoons of low-sodium soy sauce
- 1 teaspoon of ground turmeric
- 1 teaspoon of fresh lemon juice

Instructions:

1. In a frying pan, heat the vegetable oil over medium-high heat and sauté the garlic for about 1 minute
2. Add the tofu and cook for about 2-3 minutes, slowly adding the broth.

3. Add the spinach, soy, and turmeric and fry for about 3-4 minutes or until all the liquid is absorbed

4. Stir in the juice and take away from the heat.

5. Serve immediately.

Tofu & Veggie Scramble

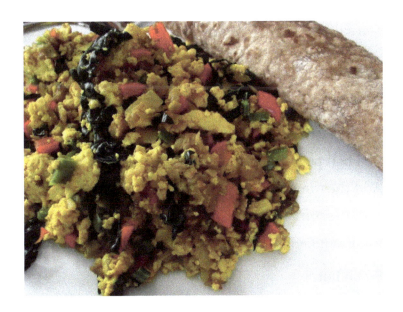

Servings: 2

Preparation Time: 15 minutes

Cooking Time: 15 minutes

Ingredients:

- ½ tablespoon of olive oil
- 1 small onion, chopped finely
- 1 small red bell pepper, seeded and chopped finely
- 1 cup of cherry tomatoes, chopped finely
- 1½ cup of firm tofu, crumbled and chopped

- Pinch of cayenne pepper
- Pinch of ground turmeric
- Sea salt, to taste

Instructions:

1. In a skillet, heat oil over medium heat and sauté the onion and bell pepper for about 4-5 minutes.
2. Add the tomatoes and cook for about 1-2 minutes.
3. Add the tofu, turmeric, cayenne pepper, and salt and cook for about 6-8 minutes.
4. Serve hot.

Apple Omelet

Servings: 1

Preparation Time: 10 minutes

Cooking Time: 9 minutes

Ingredients:

1. 2 teaspoons of olive oil, divided
2. ½ of large green apple, cored and sliced thinly
3. ¼ teaspoon of ground cinnamon
4. 1/8 teaspoon of ground nutmeg
5. 2 large eggs
6. 1/8 teaspoon of vanilla extract
7. Pinch of salt

Instructions:

1. In a non-stick frying pan, heat 1 teaspoon of oil over medium-low heat
2. Add apple slices and sprinkle with nutmeg and cinnamon.
3. Cook for about 4-5 minutes, turning once halfway through.
4. Meanwhile, in a bowl, add eggs, vanilla, and salt and beat until fluffy.
5. Add the remaining oil to the pan and let it heat completely.

6. Place the egg mixture over apple slices evenly and cook for about 3-4 minutes or until desired doneness.
7. Carefully turn the pan over a serving plate and immediately fold the omelet
8. Serve hot.

Mushroom & Tomato Omelet

Servings: 2

Preparation Time: 15 minutes

Cooking Time: 36 minutes

Ingredients:

- 2 poblano peppers
- Olive oil cooking spray
- 1 small tomato
- ½ teaspoon of dried oregano
- ½ teaspoon of chicken bouillon seasoning
- 4 eggs, separated
- 2 tablespoons of sour cream
- ½ cup of fresh white mushrooms, sliced
- 2/3 cup of part-skim mozzarella cheese, shredded and divided

Instructions:

1. Preheat your oven to the broiler.
2. Line a baking sheet with a bit of foil.
3. Spray the poblano peppers with cooking spray lightly.

4. Arrange the peppers onto the prepared baking sheet in a single layer and broil for about 5-10 minutes per side or until the skin becomes dark and blistered.
5. Remove from the oven and put aside to chill.
6. After cooking, remove the stems, skin, and seeds from peppers, then cut each into thin strips.
7. Meanwhile, for the sauce: with a knife, make 2 small slits in a crisscross pattern on the tomato's top.
8. In a microwave-safe plate, place the tomato and microwave on High for about 2-3 minutes.
9. In a blender, add the tomato, oregano, and chicken bouillon seasoning and pulse until smooth.
10. Transfer the sauce into a bowl and put it aside.
11. In a bowl, add the egg yolks and sour cream and beat until well combined.
12. In a clean glass bowl, add egg whites and with an electric mixer, beat until soft peaks form
13. Gently gold the ingredient mixture into whipped egg whites
14. Heat a lightly greased skillet over medium-low heat and cook half the egg mixture cook for about 3-5 minutes or until the bottom is about
15. Place half the mushrooms and pepper strips over the one-half omelet and sprinkle with half the cheese
16. Cover the skillet and cook for about 2-3 minutes

17. Uncover the skillet and fold in the omelet

18. Transfer the omelet onto a plate

19. Repeat with the remaining egg mixture, mushrooms, pepper strips, and cheese.

20. Top each omelet with sauce and serve.

Veggie Omelet

Servings: 4

Preparation Time: 10 minutes

Cooking Time: 25 minutes

Ingredients:

- 6 large eggs
- ½ cup of unsweetened almond milk
- Salt and ground black pepper, as required
- ½ of onion, chopped
- ¼ cup of bell pepper, seeded and chopped
- ¼ cup of fresh mushrooms, sliced
- 1 tablespoon of chives, minced

Instructions:

1. Preheat your oven to 350 degrees F.
2. Lightly grease a pie dish.
3. In a bowl, add eggs, almond milk, salt, and black pepper and beat until well combined.
4. In a separate bowl, mix onion, bell pepper, and mushrooms.

5. Place the egg mixture into the prepared pie dish evenly and top with vegetable mixture.
6. Sprinkle with chives evenly.
7. Bake for about 20-25 minutes.
8. Remove the pie dish from the oven and put it aside for about 5 minutes.
9. Cut into 4 portions and serve immediately.

Salmon & Arugula Omelet

Servings: 4

Preparation Time: 10 minutes

Cooking Time: 7 minutes

Ingredients:

- 6 eggs
- 2 tablespoons of unsweetened almond milk
- Salt and ground black pepper, as required
- 2 tablespoons of olive oil
- 4 ounces of smoked salmon, cut into bite-sized chunks
- 2 cups of fresh arugula, chopped finely
- 4 scallions, chopped finely

Instructions:

1. In a bowl, place the eggs, coconut milk, salt, and black pepper and beat well. Set aside.
2. In a non-stick skillet, heat the oil over medium heat.
3. Place the egg mixture evenly and cook for about 30 seconds without stirring.
4. Place the salmon kale and scallions on top of the egg mixture evenly.

5. Reduce heat to low and cook, covered for about 4-5 minutes or until omelet is completed completely.

6. Uncover the skillet and cook for about 1 minute.

7. Carefully transfer the omelet onto a serving plate and serve.

Tuna Omelet

Servings: 2

Preparation Time: 10 minutes

Cooking Time: 5 minutes

Ingredients:

- 4 eggs
- ¼ cup of unsweetened almond milk
- 1 tablespoon of scallions, chopped
- 1 garlic clove, minced
- ½ of jalapeño pepper, minced
- Salt and ground black pepper, to taste
- 1 (5-ounce of) can water-packed tuna, drained and flaked
- 1 tablespoon of olive oil
- 3 tablespoons of green bell pepper, seeded and chopped
- 3 tablespoons of tomato, chopped
- ¼ cup of low-fat cheddar cheese, shredded

Instructions:

1. In a bowl, add the eggs, almond milk, scallions, garlic, jalapeno, salt, and black pepper, and beat well.
2. Add the tuna and stir to mix.

3. In a large non-stick frying pan, heat oil over medium heat.
4. Place the egg mixture in a good layer and cook for about 1–2 minutes, without stirring.
5. Carefully lift the sides to run the uncooked portion flow underneath.
6. Spread the veggies over the egg mixture and sprinkle with the cheese.
7. Cover the frying pan and cook for about 30–60 seconds.
8. Remove the lid and fold the omelet in half.
9. Remove from the heat and cut the omelet into 2 portions.
10. Serve immediately.

Veggies Quiche

Servings: 4

Preparation Time: 15 minutes

Cooking Time: 25 minutes

Ingredients:

- 6 large eggs
- Salt and ground black pepper, as required
- ½ cup of unsweetened almond milk
- ½ of onion, chopped
- ¼ cup of fresh mushrooms, cut into slices
- ¼ cup of red bell pepper, seeded and diced
- 1 tablespoon of fresh chives, minced

Instructions:

1. Preheat your oven to 350 degrees F.
2. Lightly grease a pie dish.
3. In a bowl, add the eggs, salt, black pepper, and coconut oil and beat until well combined.
4. In another bowl, mix together the onion, bell pepper, and mushrooms.
5. Transfer the egg mixture into the prepared pie dish evenly.

6. Top with the vegetable mixture evenly.

7. Sprinkle with chives evenly.

8. Bake for about 20-25 minutes.

9. Remove the pie dish from the oven and put it aside for about 5 minutes.

10. Cut into equal-sized wedges and serve.

Zucchini & Carrot Quiche

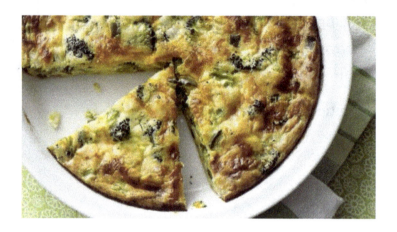

Servings: 3

Preparation Time: 10 minutes

Cooking Time: 40 minutes

Ingredients:

- 5 eggs
- Salt and ground black pepper, as required
- 1 carrot, peeled and grated
- 1 small zucchini, shredded

Instructions:

1. Preheat your oven to 350 degrees F.

2. Lightly grease the little baking dish.
3. In a large bowl, add eggs, salt, and black pepper and beat well
4. Add the carrot and zucchini and stir to mix 5. Transfer the mixture into the prepared baking dish evenly
5. Bake for about 40 minutes.
6. Remove the baking dish from the oven and put it aside for about 5 minutes.
7. Cut into equal-sized wedges and serve.

Green Veggies Quiche

Servings: 4

Preparation Time: 15 minutes

Cooking Time: 20 minutes

Ingredients:

- 6 eggs
- ½ cup of unsweetened almond milk
- Salt and ground black pepper, as required
- 2 cups of fresh baby spinach, chopped
- ½ cup of green bell pepper, seeded and chopped
- 1 scallion, chopped
- ¼ cup of fresh cilantro, chopped
- 1 tablespoon of fresh chives, minced
- 3 tablespoons of low-fat mozzarella cheese, grated

Instructions:

1. Preheat your oven to 400 degrees F.
2. Lightly grease a pie dish
3. In a large bowl, add the eggs, almond milk, salt, and black pepper and beat until well combined. Set aside.

4. In another bowl, add the vegetables and herbs and blend well.
5. In the bottom of the prepared pie dish, place the veggie mixture evenly and top with the egg mixture.
6. Bake for about 20 minutes or until a wooden skewer inserted in the center comes out clean.
7. Remove from the oven and immediately sprinkle with the Parmesan cheese.
8. put aside for about 5 minutes before slicing.
9. Cut into desired sized wedges and serve.

Chicken & Veggie Quiche

Servings: 4

Preparation Time: 15 minutes

Cooking Time: 20 minutes

Ingredients:

- 6 eggs
- ½ cup of unsweetened almond milk
- Freshly ground black pepper, to taste
- 1 cup of cooked chicken, chopped
- ½ cup of fresh baby spinach, chopped
- ½ cup of fresh baby kale, chopped
- ¼ cup of fresh mushrooms, sliced
- ¼ cup of green bell pepper, seeded and chopped
- 1 scallion, chopped
- ¼ cup of fresh cilantro, chopped
- 1 tablespoon of fresh chives, minced

Instructions:

1. Preheat the oven to 400 degrees F.

2. Lightly grease a pie dish.
3. In a large bowl, add the eggs, almond milk, salt, and black pepper and beat well. Set aside.
4. In another bowl, add the chicken, vegetables, scallion, and herbs and blend well.
5. Place the chicken mixture in the bottom of the prepared pie dish.
6. Place the egg mixture over the chicken mixture evenly.
7. Bake for about 20 minutes or until a toothpick inserted in the center comes out clean.
8. Remove from the oven and put aside to chill for about 5-10 minutes before slicing.
9. Cut into desired size wedges and serve.

Kale & Mushroom Frittata

Servings: 5

Preparation Time: 15 minutes

Cooking Time: 30 minutes

Ingredients:

- 8 eggs
- ½ cup of unsweetened almond milk
- Salt and ground black pepper, as required
- 1 tablespoon of extra-virgin olive oil
- 1 onion, chopped
- 1 garlic clove, minced
- 1 cup of fresh mushrooms, chopped
- 1½ cup of fresh kale, tough ribs removed, and chopped

Instructions:

1. Preheat your oven to 350 degrees F.
2. Place the eggs, almond milk, salt, and black pepper in a large bowl and beat well. Set aside.
3. In a large ovenproof wok, heat the oil over medium heat and sauté the onion and garlic for about 3-4 minutes.

4. Add the mushrooms, kale, salt, and black pepper and cook for about 8-10 minutes.
5. Stir in the mushrooms and cook for about 3-4 minutes.
6. Add the kale and cook for about 5 minutes.
7. Place the egg mixture on top evenly and cook for about 4 minutes, without stirring.
8. Transfer the wok to the oven and Bake for about 12-15 minutes or until desired doneness.
9. Remove from the oven and place the frittata side for about 3-5 minutes before serving.
10. Cut into desired sized wedges and serve.

Kale & Bell Pepper Frittata

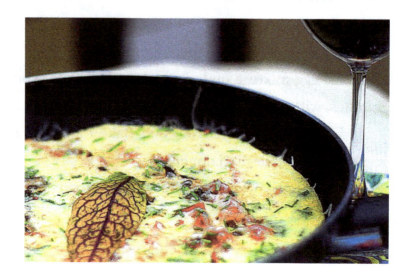

Servings: 3

Preparation Time: 10 minutes

Cooking Time: 17 minutes

Ingredients:

- 6 eggs
- Salt, as required
- 1 tablespoon of olive oil
- ½ teaspoon of ground turmeric
- 1 small red bell pepper, seeded and chopped
- 1 cup of fresh kale, trimmed and chopped

- ¼ cup of fresh chives, chopped

Instructions:

1. In a bowl, add the eggs and salt and beat well. Set aside.
2. In a cast-iron skillet, heat the oil over medium-low heat and sprinkle with turmeric.
3. Immediately stir in the bell pepper and kale and sauté for about 2 minutes.
4. Place the beaten eggs over the bell pepper mixture evenly and immediately reduce the heat to low.
5. Cover the skillet and cook for about 10-15 minutes.
6. Remove from the heat and put aside for about 5 minutes.
7. Cut into equal-sized wedges and serve.

Bell Pepper Frittata

Servings: 6

Preparation Time: 15 minutes

Cooking Time: 10 minutes

Ingredients:

- 8 eggs
- 1 tablespoon of fresh cilantro, chopped
- 1 tablespoon of fresh basil, chopped
- ¼ teaspoon of red pepper flakes, crushed
- Salt and ground black pepper, as required
- 2 tablespoons of olive oil
- 1 bunch scallions, chopped
- 1 cup of bell pepper, seeded and sliced thinly
- ½ cup of goat cheese, crumbled

Instructions:

1. Preheat the broiler of the oven.
2. Arrange a rack in the upper third of the oven.
3. In a bowl, add the eggs, fresh herbs, red pepper flakes, salt, and black pepper and beat well.

4. In an ovenproof skillet, heat the oil over medium heat and sauté the scallion and bell pepper for about 1 minute.

5. Add the egg mixture over the bell pepper mixture evenly, lift the sides to let the egg mixture flow underneath, and cook for about 2-3 minutes.

1. 6 Place the cheese on top in the sort of dots.

6. Now, transfer the skillet under broiler and broil for about 2-3 minutes.

7. Remove from the oven and put aside for about 5 minutes before serving.

8. Cut the frittata into desired sized slices and serve.

Broccoli Frittata

Servings: 6

Preparation Time: 15 minutes

Cooking Time: 13 minutes

Ingredients:

- 8 eggs
- 1 tablespoon of fresh cilantro, chopped
- 1 tablespoon of fresh basil, chopped
- ¼ teaspoon of red pepper flakes, crushed
- Salt and ground black pepper, as required
- 2 tablespoons of olive oil
- 1 bunch scallions, chopped
- 1 cup of broccoli, chopped finely
- ½ cup of goat cheese, crumbled

Instructions:

1. Preheat the broiler of the oven.
2. Arrange a rack in the upper third of the oven.
3. In a bowl, add eggs, fresh herbs, red pepper flakes, salt, and black pepper and beat well.

4. In an ovenproof skillet, heat the oil over medium heat and sauté scallion and broccoli for about 1-2 minutes.

5. Add the egg mixture over the broccoli mixture evenly and lift the sides to let the egg mixture flow underneath.

6. Cook for about 2-3 minutes.

7. Place the cheese on top in the type of dots.

8. Now, transfer the skillet under broiler and broil for about 2-3 minutes.

9. Remove the skillet from the oven and put it aside for about 5 minutes.

10. Cut the frittata into desired size slices and serve.

Zucchini Frittata

Servings: 6

Preparation Time: 15 minutes

Cooking Time: 20 minutes

Ingredients:

- 2 tablespoons of unsweetened almond milk
- 8 eggs
- Freshly ground black pepper, to taste
- 1 tablespoon of olive oil
- 1 garlic clove, minced
- 2 medium zucchinis, cut into ¼-inch thick round slices
- ½ cup of goat cheese, crumbled

Instructions:

1. Preheat the oven to 350 degrees F.
2. In a bowl, add the almond milk, eggs, and black pepper, and black pepper and beat well.
3. In an ovenproof skillet, heat the oil over medium heat and sauté the garlic for about 1 minute.
4. Stir in the zucchini and cook for about 5 minutes.
5. Add the egg mixture and stir for about 1 minute.

6. Sprinkle the cheese on top evenly.

7. Immediately transfer the skillet into the oven.

8. Bake for about 12 minutes or until eggs become set. 9. Remove from oven and put aside to chill for about 5 minutes.

9. Cut into desired size wedges and serve.

Chicken & Asparagus Frittata

Servings: 4

Preparation Time: 15 minutes

Cooking Time: 12 minutes

Ingredients:

- ½ cup of cooked chicken, chopped
- 1/3 cup of low-fat Parmesan cheese, grated
- 6 eggs, beaten lightly
- Salt and ground black pepper, as required
- 1 teaspoon of coconut oil
- ½ cup of boiled asparagus, chopped
- 1 tablespoon of fresh parsley, chopped

Instructions:

1. Preheat the broiler of the oven.
2. In a bowl, add the cheese, eggs, salt, and black pepper and beat until well combined.
3. In a large ovenproof skillet, melt coconut oil over medium-high heat and cook the chicken and asparagus for about 2-3 minutes.
4. Add the egg mixture and stir to mix,

5. Cook for about 4-5 minutes.
6. Remove from the heat and sprinkle with the parsley.
7. Now, transfer the skillet under broiler and broil for about 3-4 minutes or until slightly puffed.
8. Cut into desired sized wedges and serve immediately.

Chicken & Veggie Frittata

Servings: 8

Preparation Time: 45 minutes

Cooking Time: 15 minutes

Ingredients:

- 1 teaspoon of olive oil
- ½ cup of yellow onion, sliced
- 2 garlic cloves, minced
- 2 cups of fresh spinach, chopped
- 1 cup of red bell pepper, seeded and chopped
- 2 cups of cooked chicken, chopped
- 2 large eggs
- 4 large egg whites
- 1¼ cup of unsweetened almond milk
- 1 cup of low-fat cheddar cheese, shredded
- Freshly ground black pepper, as required
- 1 tablespoon of Parmesan cheese, shredded

Instructions:

1. Preheat your oven to 350 degrees F.
2. Grease a 9-inch pie plate.

3. In a skillet, heat oil over medium heat and sauté onion and garlic for about 2-3 minutes.
4. Add spinach and bell pepper and sauté for about 1-2 minutes.
5. Stir in chicken and transfer the mixture into the prepared pie dish evenly.
6. Add eggs, egg whites, almond milk, cheddar, salt, and black pepper in a bowl and beat until well combined.
7. Pour egg mixture over the chicken mixture evenly and top with Parmesan cheese.
8. Bake for about 40 minutes or until the top becomes golden brown.
9. Remove the pie dish from the oven and put aside for about 5 minutes.
10. Cut into 8 equal-sized wedges and serve.

Eggs with Spinach

Servings: 2

Preparation Time: 10 minutes

Cooking Time: 22 minutes

Ingredients:

- 6 cup of fresh baby spinach
- 2-3 tablespoons of water
- 4 eggs
- Salt and ground black pepper, as required
- 2-3 tablespoons of feta cheese, crumbled

Instructions:

1. Preheat your oven to 400 degrees F.
2. Lightly grease 2 small baking dishes.
3. In a large frying pan, add spinach and water over medium heat and cook for about 3-4 minutes.
4. Remove the frying pan from heat and drain the surplus water completely.
5. Divide the spinach into prepared baking dishes evenly.
6. Carefully crack 2 eggs in each baking dish over spinach.

7. Sprinkle with salt and black pepper and top with feta cheese evenly.

8. Arrange the baking dishes onto a large cooking utensil.

9. Bake for about 15-18 minutes.

10. Serve warm.

Eggs with Kale & Tomatoes

Servings: 4

Preparation Time: 15 minutes

Cooking Time: 25 minutes

Ingredients:

- 2 tablespoons of olive oil
- 1 yellow onion, chopped
- 2 garlic cloves, minced
- 1 cup of tomatoes, chopped
- ½ pound fresh kale, tough ribs removed and chopped
- 1 teaspoon of ground cumin
- ¼ teaspoon of red pepper flakes, crushed
- Salt and ground black pepper, as required
- 4 eggs
- 2 tablespoons of fresh parsley, chopped

Instructions:

1. In a large non-stick wok, heat the olive oil over medium heat and sauté the onion for about 4-5 minutes.
2. Add in the garlic and sauté for about 1 minute.

3. Add the tomatoes, spices, salt, and black pepper and cook for about 2-3 minutes, stirring frequently.

4. Add in the kale and cook for about 4-5 minutes.

5. Carefully crack eggs on top of the kale mixture.

6. With the lid, cover the wok and cook for about 10 minutes or until the eggs' desired doneness.

7. Serve hot with the garnishing of parsley.

Eggs with Veggies

Servings: 4

Preparation Time: 10 minutes

Cooking Time: 15 minutes

Ingredients:

- 2 tablespoons of olive oil, divided
- ¾ pound zucchini, quartered and sliced thinly
- 1 red bell pepper, seeded and chopped
- 1 medium onion, chopped
- 1 teaspoon of fresh rosemary, chopped finely
- Salt and ground black pepper, as required
- 4 large eggs

Instructions:

1. In a large skillet, heat 1 tablespoon of oil over medium-high heat and sauté the zucchini, bell pepper, and onion for about 5-8 minutes.
2. Add the rosemary, salt, and black pepper and stir to mix.
3. With a wooden spoon, make a large well in the center of the skillet by moving the veggie mixture towards the edges.

4. Reduce the heat to medium and pour the remaining oil into the well.
5. Carefully crack the eggs in the well and sprinkle the eggs with salt and black pepper.
6. Cook for about 1-2 minutes.
7. Cover the skillet and cook for about 1-2 minutes more.
8. For serving, carefully scoop the veggie mixture onto 4 serving plates.
9. Top each serving with an egg and serve.

Chicken & Zucchini Muffins

Servings: 4

Preparation Time: 15 minutes

Cooking Time: 15 minutes

Ingredients:

- 4 eggs
- ¼ cup of olive oil
- ¼ cup of water
- 1/3 cup of coconut flour
- ½ teaspoon of baking powder
- ¼ teaspoon of salt
- ¾ cup of cooked chicken, shredded
- ¾ cup of zucchini, grated
- ½ cup of low-fat Parmesan cheese, shredded
- 1 tablespoon of fresh oregano, minced
- 1 tablespoon of fresh thyme, minced
- ¼ cup of low-fat cheddar cheese, grated

Instructions:

1. Preheat your oven to 400 degrees F.
2. Lightly grease 8 cups of a muffin pan.

3. In a bowl, add eggs, oil, and water and beat until well combined

4. Add the flour, baking powder, and salt, and blend well.

5. Add the remaining ingredients and blend until just combined.

6. Place the muffin mixture into the prepared muffin cup evenly.

   Bake for about 13-15 minutes or until tops become golden brown.

8. Remove muffin pan from oven and place onto a wire rack to chill for about 10 minutes.

9. Invert the muffins onto a platter and serve warm.

Chicken & Bell Pepper Muffins

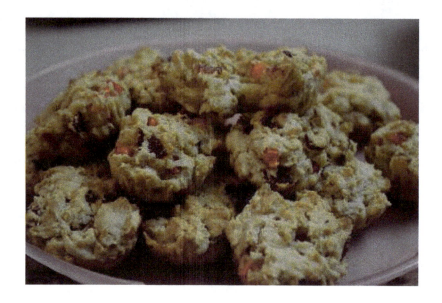

Servings: 4

Preparation Time: 15 minutes

Cooking Time: 20 minutes

Ingredients:

- 8 eggs
- Salt and ground black pepper, as required
- 2 tablespoons of water
- 8 ounces of cooked chicken, chopped finely
- 1 cup of green bell pepper, seeded and chopped

- 1 cup of onion, chopped

Instructions:

1. Preheat your oven to 350 degrees F.
2. Grease 8 cups of a muffin tin.
3. In a bowl, add eggs, black pepper, and water and beat until well combined.
4. Add the chicken, bell pepper, and onion and stir to mix.
5. Transfer the mixture to the prepared muffin cup evenly.
6. Bake for about 18-20 minutes or until golden brown.
7. Remove the muffin tin from the oven and place onto a wire rack to chill for about 10 minutes.
8. Carefully invert the muffins onto a platter and serve warm.

Chicken & Kale Muffins

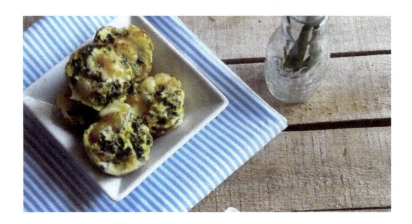

Servings: 4

Preparation Time: 15 minutes

Cooking Time: 20 minutes

Ingredients:

- 8 eggs
- Freshly ground black pepper, as required
- 2 tablespoons of water
- 7 ounces of cooked chicken, chopped finely
- 1½ cup of fresh kale, tough ribs removed, and chopped
- 1 cup of onion, chopped
- 2 tablespoons of fresh parsley, chopped

Instructions:

1. Preheat your oven to 350 degrees F.
2. Grease 8 cups of a muffin tin.
3. In a bowl, add eggs, black pepper, and water and beat until well combined.
4. Add chicken, kale, onion, and parsley and stir to mix.
5. Transfer the mixture in the prepared muffin cup evenly.
6. Bake for about 18-20 minutes or until golden brown.
7. Remove the muffin tin from the oven and place onto a wire rack to chill for about 10 minutes.
8. Carefully invert the muffins onto a platter and serve warm.

Chicken & Zucchini Muffins

Servings: 4

Preparation Time: 15 minutes

Cooking Time: 15 minutes

Ingredients:

- 4 eggs
- ¼ cup of olive oil
- ¼ cup of water
- 1/3 cup of coconut flour
- ½ teaspoon of baking powder
- ¼ teaspoon of salt
- ¾ cup of cooked chicken, shredded
- ¾ cup of zucchini, grated
- ½ cup of low-fat Parmesan cheese, shredded
- 1 tablespoon of fresh oregano, minced
- 1 tablespoon of fresh thyme, minced
- ¼ cup of low-fat cheddar cheese, grated

Instructions:

1. Preheat your oven to 400 degrees F.

2. Lightly grease 8 cups of a muffin pan.

3. In a bowl, add eggs, oil, water, and beat until well combined.

4. Add the flour, baking powder, and salt, and blend well.

5. Add the remaining ingredients and blend until just combined.

6. Place the muffin mixture into the prepared muffin cup of evenly.

7. Bake for about 13–15 minutes or until tops become golden brown.

8. Remove muffin pan from oven and place onto a wire rack to chill for about 10 minutes.

9. Invert the muffins onto a platter and serve warm.

Tofu & Mushroom Muffins

Servings: 6

Preparation Time: 15 minutes

Cooking Time: 30 minutes

Ingredients:

- 2 teaspoons of olive oil, divided
- 1½ cups of fresh mushrooms, chopped
- 1 scallion, chopped
- 1 teaspoon of garlic, minced
- 1 teaspoon of fresh rosemary, minced
- Freshly ground black pepper, as required
- 1 (12.3-ounce of) package lite firm silken tofu, drained
- ¼ cup of unsweetened almond milk
- 2 tablespoons of nutritional yeast
- 1 tablespoon of arrowroot starch
- ¼ teaspoon of ground turmeric

Instructions:

1. Preheat your oven to 375 degrees F.
2. Grease 12 cups of muffin tin.

3. In a non-stick skillet, heat 1 teaspoon of oil over medium heat and sauté scallion and garlic for about 1 minute.

4. Add mushrooms and sauté for about 5-7 minutes.

5. Stir in the rosemary and black pepper and take away from the heat.

6. Put aside to chill slightly.

7. In a food processor, add tofu and remaining ingredients and pulse until smooth.

8. Transfer the tofu mixture into a large bowl

9. Fold in mushroom mixture.

10. Transfer the mixture into the prepared muffin cup of evenly.

11. Bake for about 20-22 minutes or until a toothpick inserted in the center comes out clean.

12. Remove the muffin pan from the oven and place it onto a wire rack to chill for about 10 minutes.

13. Carefully invert the muffins onto the wire rack and serve warm.

Fruit Salad

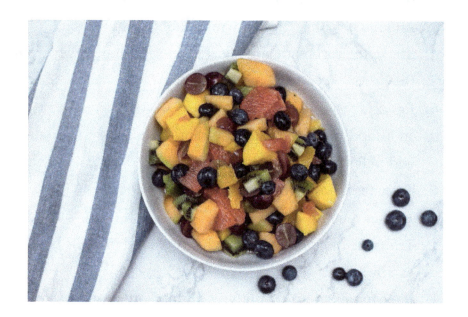

Servings: 4

Preparation Time: 15 minutes

Ingredients:

For Salad

- 4 cups of fresh baby arugula
- 1 cup of fresh strawberries, hulled and sliced
- 2 oranges, peeled and segmented

For Dressing

- 2 tablespoons of fresh lemon juice
- 2-3 drops liquid stevia
- 2 teaspoons of extra-virgin olive oil
- Salt and ground black pepper, as required

Instructions:

1. For Salad: in a salad bowl, place all ingredients and blend.
2. For Dressing: Place all ingredients in another bowl and beat until well combined.
3. Place dressing on top of the Salad and toss to coat well.
4. Serve immediately.

Strawberry, Orange & Rocket Salad

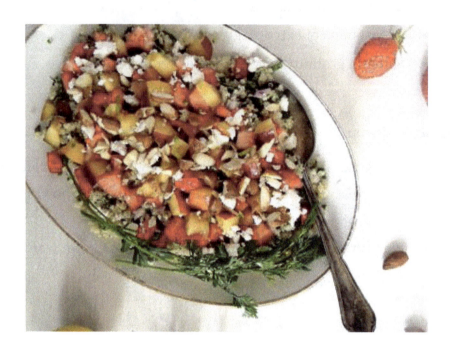

Servings: 4

Preparation Time: 15 minutes

Ingredients:

For Salad:

- 6 cups of fresh rocket
- 1½ cups of fresh strawberries, hulled and sliced
- 2 oranges, peeled and segmented

For Dressing:

- 2 tablespoons of fresh lemon juice
- 1 tablespoon of raw honey
- 2 teaspoons of extra-virgin olive oil
- 1 teaspoon of Dijon mustard
- Salt and ground black pepper, as required

Instructions:

1. For Salad: in a salad bowl, place all ingredients and blend.
2. For Dressing: Place all ingredients in another bowl and beat until well combined.
3. Place dressing on top of the Salad and toss to coat well.
4. Serve immediately.

Strawberry & Asparagus Salad

Servings: 8

Preparation Time: 15 minutes

Cooking Time: 5 minutes

Ingredients:

- 2 pounds fresh asparagus, trimmed and sliced
- 3 cups of fresh strawberries, hulled and sliced
- ¼ cup of extra-virgin olive oil
- ¼ cup of balsamic vinegar
- 2 tablespoons of maple syrup
- Salt and ground black pepper, as required

Instructions:

1. In a pan of water, add the asparagus over medium-high heat and bring to a boil.
2. Boil the asparagus for about 2-3 minutes or until hard.
3. Drain the asparagus and immediately transfer it into a bowl of drinking water to chill completely.
4. Drain the asparagus and pat dry with paper towels.
5. In a large bowl, add the asparagus and strawberries and blend.

6. In a small bowl, add the vegetable oil, vinegar, honey, salt, and black pepper and beat until well blended.

7. Place the dressing over the asparagus strawberry mixture and gently toss to coat.

8. Refrigerate for about 1 hour before serving.

Blueberries & Spinach Salad

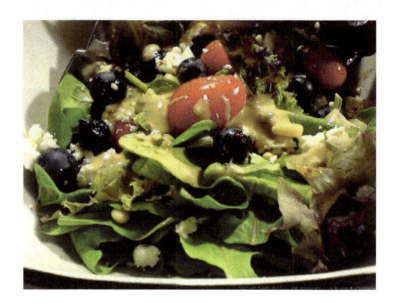

Servings: 4

Preparation Time: 15 minutes

Ingredients:

For Salad:

- 6 cups of fresh baby spinach
- 1½ cup of fresh blueberries
- ¼ cup of onion, sliced
- ¼ cup of almond, sliced
- ¼ cup of feta cheese, crumbled

For Dressing:

- 1/3 cup of olive oil
- 2 tablespoons of fresh lemon juice
- ¼ teaspoon of liquid stevia
- 1/8 teaspoon of garlic powder Salt, as required

Instructions:

1. For Salad: In a bowl, add the spinach, berries, onion, and almonds and blend.
2. For Dressing: in another small bowl, add all the ingredients and beat until well blended.
3. Place the dressing over Salad and gently toss to coat well.
4. Serve immediately.

Mixed Berries Salad

Servings: 4

Preparation Time: 15 minutes

Ingredients:

- 1 cup of fresh strawberries, hulled and sliced
- ½ cups of fresh blackberries
- ½ cup of fresh blueberries
- ½ cup of fresh raspberries
- 6 cup of fresh arugula
- 2 tablespoons of extra-virgin olive oil
- Salt and ground black pepper, as required

Instructions:

1. In a salad bowl, place all the ingredients and toss to coat well.
2. Serve immediately.

Kale & Citrus Fruit Salad

Servings: 2

Preparation Time: 15 minutes

Ingredients:

For Salad:

- 3 cups of fresh kale, tough ribs removed and torn
- 1 orange, peeled and segmented
- 1 grapefruit, peeled and segmented
- 2 tablespoons of unsweetened dried cranberries
- ¼ teaspoon of white sesame seeds

For Dressing:

- 2 tablespoons of extra-virgin olive oil
- 2 tablespoons of fresh orange juice
- 1 teaspoon of Dijon mustard
- ½ teaspoon of raw honey
- Salt and ground black pepper, as required

Instructions:

1. For Salad: in a salad bowl, place all ingredients and blend.

2. For Dressing: Place all ingredients in another bowl and beat until well combined.

3. Place dressing on top of the Salad and toss to coat well.

4. Serve immediately.

Kale, Apple & Cranberry Salad

Servings: 4

Preparation Time: 15 minutes

Ingredients:

- 6 cups of fresh baby kale
- 3 large apples, cored and sliced
- ¼ cup of unsweetened dried cranberries
- ¼ cup of almonds, sliced
- 2 tablespoons of extra-virgin olive oil
- 1 tablespoon of raw honey
- Salt and ground black pepper, as required

Instructions:

1. In a salad bowl, place all the ingredients and toss to coat well.
2. Serve immediately.

Rocket, Beat & Orange Salad

Servings: 4

Preparation Time: 15 minutes

Ingredients:

- 3 large oranges, peeled, seeded, and sectioned
- 2 beets, trimmed, peeled, and sliced
- 6 cups of fresh rocket
- ¼ cup of walnuts, chopped
- 3 tablespoons of olive oil Pinch of salt

Instructions:

1. In a salad bowl, place all ingredients and gently toss to coat.
2. Serve immediately.

Cucumber & Tomato Salad

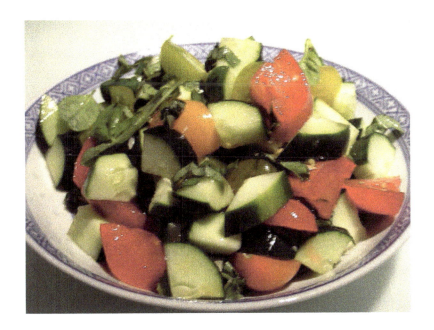

Servings: 6

Preparation Time: 15 minutes

Ingredients:

For Salad:

- 3 large English cucumbers, sliced thinly sliced
- 2 cups of tomatoes, chopped
- 6 cup of lettuce, torn

For Dressing:

- 4 tablespoons of olive oil
- 2 tablespoons of balsamic vinegar
- 1 tablespoon of fresh lemon juice
- Salt and ground black pepper, as required

Instructions:

1. For Salad: In a large bowl, add the cucumbers, onion, and dill and blend.
2. For Dressing: In a small bowl, add all the ingredients and beat until well combined.
3. Place the dressing over the Salad and toss to coat well.
4. Serve immediately.

Mixed Veggie Salad

Servings: 6

Preparation Time: 20 minutes

Ingredients:

For Dressing:

- 1 small avocado, peeled, pitted, and chopped
- ¼ cup of low-fat plain Greek yogurt
- 1 small yellow onion, chopped
- 1 garlic clove, chopped
- 2 tablespoons of fresh parsley
- 2 tablespoons of fresh lemon juice

For Salad:

- 6 cups of fresh spinach, shredded
- Two medium zucchinis, cut into thin slices
- ½ cup of celery, sliced
- ½ cup of red bell pepper, seeded and sliced thinly
- ½ cup of yellow onion, sliced thinly
- ½ cup of cucumber, sliced thinly
- ½ cup of cherry tomatoes halved
- ¼ cup of Kalamata olives pitted
- ½ cup of feta cheese, crumbled

Instructions:

1. For Dressing: In a food processor, add all the ingredients and pulse until smooth.
2. For Salad: In a salad bowl, add all the ingredients and blend well.
3. Pour the dressing over Salad and gently toss to coat well.
4. Serve immediately.

Eggs & Veggie Salad

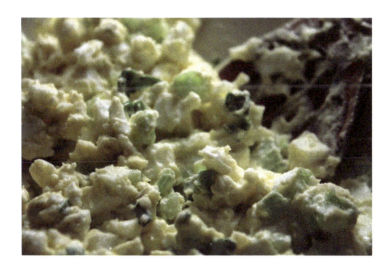

Servings: 8

Preparation Time: 15 minutes

Ingredients:

For Salad:

- 2 large English cucumbers, sliced thinly sliced
- 2 cups of tomatoes, chopped
- 8 hard-boiled eggs, peeled and sliced
- 8 cups of fresh baby spinach

For Dressing:

- 4 tablespoons of olive oil

- 2 tablespoons of balsamic vinegar
- 1 tablespoon of fresh lemon juice
- Salt and ground black pepper, as required

Instructions:

1. For Salad: In a salad bowl, add the cucumbers, onion, and dill and blend.
2. For Dressing: In a small bowl, add all the ingredients and beat until well blended.
3. Place the dressing over the Salad and toss to coat well.
4. Serve immediately.

Chicken & Orange Salad

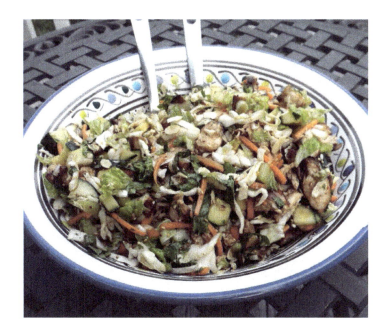

Servings: 5

Preparation Time: 15 minutes

Cooking Time: 16 minutes

Ingredients:

For Chicken:

- 4 (6-ounce of) boneless, skinless chicken breast halves
- Salt and ground black pepper, as required
- 2 tablespoons of extra-virgin olive oil

95

For Salad:

- 8 cups of fresh baby arugula
- 5 medium oranges, peeled and sectioned
- 1 cup of onion, sliced

For Dressing:

- 2 tablespoons of extra-virgin olive oil
- 2 tablespoons of fresh orange juice
- 2 tablespoons of balsamic vinegar
- 1½ teaspoons of shallots, minced
- 1 garlic clove, minced
- Salt and ground black pepper, as required

Instructions:

1. For chicken: season each chicken breast half with salt and black pepper evenly.
2. Place chicken over a rack set in a rimmed baking sheet.
3. Refrigerate for at least 30 minutes.
4. Remove the baking sheet from the refrigerator and pat dry the chicken breast halves with paper towels.
5. Heat the oil in a 12-inch sauté pan over medium-low heat.
6. Place the chicken breast halves, smooth-side down, and cook for about 9-10 minutes, without moving.

7. Flip the chicken breasts and cook for about 6 minutes or until cooked through.

8. Remove the sauté pan from heat and let the chicken substitute the pan for about 3 minutes.

9. Transfer the chicken breasts onto a chopping board for about 5 minutes.

10. Cut each chicken breast half into desired-sized slices.

11. For Salad: Place all ingredients in a salad bowl and blend.

12. Add chicken slices and stir to mix.

13. For Dressing: Place all ingredients in another bowl and beat until well combined.

14. Place the Salad onto each serving plate.

15. Drizzle with dressing and serve.

Chicken & Strawberry Salad

Servings: 8

Preparation Time: 20 minutes

Cooking Time: 16 minutes

Ingredients:

- 2 pounds boneless, skinless chicken breasts
- ½ cup of olive oil
- ¼ cup of fresh lemon juice 2 tablespoons of Erythritol
- 1 garlic clove, minced
- Salt and ground black pepper, as required
- 4 cups of fresh strawberries
- 8 cups of fresh spinach, torn

Instructions:

1. For marinade: In a large bowl, add oil, lime juice, Erythritol, garlic, salt, and black pepper, and beat until well combined.
2. In a large resealable bag, place chicken and ¾ cup of marinade.
3. Seal bag and shake to coat well.
4. Refrigerate overnight.

5. Cover the bowl of remaining marinade and refrigerate before serving.
6. Preheat the grill to medium heat. Grease the grill grate.
7. Remove the chicken from the bag and discard the marinade.
8. Place the chicken onto grill grate and grill, covered for about 5-8 minutes per side.
9. Remove chicken from the grill and cut into bite-sized pieces.
10. In a large bowl, add the chicken pieces, strawberries, and spinach and blend.
11. Place the reserved marinade and toss to coat.
12. Serve immediately.

Chicken & Fruit Salad

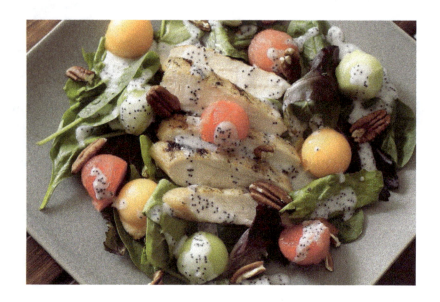

Servings: 4

Preparation Time: 15 minutes

Ingredients:

For Vinaigrette:

- 2 tablespoons of apple cider vinegar
- 2 tablespoons of extra-virgin olive oil
- Salt and freshly ground black pepper, to taste

For Salad:

- 2 cup of cooked chicken, cubed

- 4 cup of lettuce, torn
- 1 large apple, peeled, cored, and chopped
- 1 cup of fresh strawberries, hulled and sliced

Instructions:

1. For vinaigrette: In a small bowl, add all ingredients and beat well.
2. For Salad: In a large salad bowl, mix all ingredients.
3. Place vinaigrette over chicken mixture and toss to coat well.
4. Serve immediately.

Chicken, Tomato & Arugula Salad

Servings: 4

Preparation Time: 15 minutes

Cooking Time: 15 minutes

Ingredients:

For Chicken:

- 3 (6-ounce of) skinless, boneless chicken breast halves
- 2 teaspoons of orange zest, grated finely
- 1/3 cup of fresh orange juice
- 4 garlic cloves, minced
- 2 tablespoons of maple syrup
- 1½ teaspoons of dried thyme, crushed

For Salad:

- 6 cups of fresh baby arugula
- 2 cups of cherry tomatoes, quartered
- 3 tablespoons of extra-virgin olive oil
- 2 tablespoons of fresh lime juice
- Salt and ground black pepper, as required

Instructions:

1. For chicken: in a zip lock bag, all the ingredients.
2. Seal the bag and shake to coat well.
3. Refrigerate to marinate for about 6-8 hours, flipping occasionally.
4. Preheat the oven to the broiler.
5. Line a broiler pan with a bit of foil.
6. Arrange the oven rack about 6-inch far away from the heating element.
7. Remove the chicken breasts from the bag and discard the marinade.
8. Arrange the chicken breasts onto the prepared pan in a single layer.
9. Broil for about 15 minutes, flipping once halfway through.
10. Remove the chicken breasts from the oven and place onto a chopping board for about 10 minutes.
11. Cut the chicken breasts into desired sized slices.
12. For Salad: In a bowl, add all ingredients and toss to coat well.
13. Add chicken slices and stir to mix.
14. Serve immediately.

Chicken, Cucumber & Tomato Salad

Servings: 4

Preparation Time: 15 minutes

Cooking Time: 16 minutes

Ingredients:

- 4 (6-ounce of) boneless, skinless chicken breast halves
- Salt and freshly ground black pepper, to taste
- 2 tablespoons of olive oil
- 1 tomato, chopped
- 1 cucumber, chopped
- 3 cup of fresh baby greens
- 3 cup of lettuce, torn

Instructions:

1. Season each chicken breast half with salt and black pepper evenly.
2. Place chicken over a rack set in a rimmed baking sheet.
3. Refrigerate for at least 30 minutes.
4. Remove from refrigerator and with paper towels, pat dry the chicken breasts.
5. In a 12-inch skillet, heat the oil over medium-low heat.

6. Place the chicken breast halves, smooth-side down, and cook for about 9-10 minutes, without moving.

7. Flip the chicken breasts and cook for about 6 minutes or until cooked through.

8. Remove the skillet from heat and let the chicken substitute the pan for about 3 minutes.

9. Divide greens, lettuce, cucumber, and tomatoes onto serving plates.

10. Top each plate with 1 breast half and serve.

Chicken, Kale & Olives Salad

Servings: 4

Preparation Time: 15 minutes

Ingredients:

For Dressing:

- 2 tablespoons of fresh orange juice
- 2 tablespoons of fresh lemon juice
- 3 tablespoons of extra-virgin olive oil
- 1 tablespoon of red wine vinegar
- 1 tablespoon of honey
- 1 tablespoon of fresh orange zest, grated
- ¾ tablespoon of Dijon mustard
- Salt and ground black pepper, as required

For Salad:

- 3 cups of cooked chicken, chopped
- 2 cups of mixed olives, pitted
- 1 cup of red onion, chopped
- 6 cups of fresh kale, tough ribs removed and torn

Instructions:

1. For Dressing: In a small bowl, add all ingredients and beat well.
2. For Salad: In a large salad bowl, mix all ingredients.
3. Place dressing over Salad and toss to coat well.
4. Serve immediately.

Printed in the USA
CPSIA information can be obtained
at www.ICGtesting.com
LVHW021505151023
761145LV00013B/965